To God Almighty,

In the vast expanse of the universe, I humbly dedicate this ebook to the divine force that guides our paths, grants us wisdom, and blesses us with the capacity to transform our lives through the power of mindset.

To Lovina Donatus, my love,

Your unwavering support, love, and encouragement have been the driving force behind this endeavor. Your belief in me has illuminated the path of the Holistic Self-Care. This ebook is a tribute to the love and inspiration you bring into my life every day.

To my family for support,

To my family, whose love, understanding, and encouragement have been my steadfast foundation. Your belief in my journey and the principles I embrace has been a source of strength and motivation.

To everyone who desires a change of mindset,

This ebook is dedicated to each and every soul who aspires to break free from limiting beliefs, embrace growth, and embark on a transformational journey. May the wisdom contained within these pages serve as a beacon of hope and empowerment, lighting the way to a new mindset, a brighter future, and boundless possibilities.

With gratitude and profound dedication,

Chimezie Igwe

"Self-care is not a luxury; it's a necessity. It's a conscious choice to honor the temple that houses your mind, nourish the vessel that carries your spirit, and create harmony between the body and soul."

CHIMEZIE IGWE

CONTENTS

PREFACE

Welcome to the journey of self-discovery and well-being through the pages of "Holistic Self-Care: Balancing Mind, Body, and Spirit." In these transformative chapters, we embark on a voyage that delves into the intricate and interconnected facets of your holistic well-being.

This eBook is not just a collection of words; it's a roadmap to nurturing the essence of who you are. It's an exploration of mindfulness practices that calm the chaos of the mind, a guide to nutrition that nourishes the body, a journey into physical wellness that invigorates your being, and a quest for spirituality that feeds the soul.

The concept of holistic self-care recognizes that you are more than the sum of your parts. You are the thoughts that dance in your mind, the sensations that pulse through your body, and the yearnings that stir your spirit. This eBook is an invitation to honor and celebrate the totality of your existence.

Within these pages, you'll find practical guidance, inspiring stories, and a wealth of resources to support your holistic self-care journey. From the art of mindfulness meditation to the science of nutrition, from the joy of movement to the depths of spirituality, we will explore the tools and practices that empower you to thrive.

As you read through these chapters, I encourage you to approach them with an open heart and an open mind. Your journey toward holistic well-being is deeply personal, and there is no one-size-fits-all approach. Take what resonates with you, adapt it to your unique needs, and allow it to flourish within your life.

This eBook is not a destination but a path—one that you walk at your own pace, guided by your intuition and desires. It is a commitment to self-care, a pledge to prioritize your well-being, and a celebration of the magnificent tapestry of your existence.

I invite you to turn the page and begin this journey with an open heart, for within these words lie the potential for transformation, balance, and the profound embrace of your own holistic well-being.

With warm regards,

Chimezie Igwe

INTRODUCTION

It's a pleasure to welcome you to "Holistic Self-Care: Balancing Mind, Body, and Spirit." The pressures on our time and energy are constant in the fast-paced, connected society we live in today. We balance our objectives and dreams with our employment, families, relationships, and other duties. We frequently forget about the most crucial component of our lives when caught up in this whirlwind: ourselves.

This eBook will help you rediscover the art of self-care as a necessary requirement for a happy and balanced life, not as a luxury. It invites you to set out on a transformative journey that acknowledges the complex interactions between your mind, body, and spirit and gives you the tools to give each of these aspects the attention and care they need.

THE IMPORTANCE OF HOLISTIC SELF-CARE

The theory and practice of holistic self-care recognize the irrefutable connection between our physical, mental, and spiritual health. It recognizes that concentrating only on one facet of ourselves will not lead to true well-being. Instead, it necessitates a unified and thorough strategy that incorporates all aspects of our existence.

Think about it: Your body's health is influenced by your mind, which is where your thoughts and emotions originate. Your physical health has an impact on how clear your thinking is. And your spirit, the core of your inner self, is closely related to your intellect and body. It's a fine dance, and if one part is missed, the whole piece suffers.

THE JOURNEY BEGINS

You will go on a path of self-discovery and empowerment as you navigate these pages. It will provide you with the information and resources you need to improve your mental sharpness, support your physical vigor, and feed your spiritual nature. The goal is to help you thrive in every element of life; not merely assist you in dealing with its responsibilities.

This eBook is neither a panacea nor a one-size-fits-all method. Instead, it is a comprehensive framework that values your individuality. It pushes you to explore and try new things in order to discover what truly speaks to your inner being. It honors your independence in creating a self-care routine that fits your own requirements and goals.

WHAT TO EXPECT

We will go into great detail on the three components of holistic self-care—the mind, the body, and the spirit—in the chapters that follow. You will learn the skill of mindfulness and stress reduction, as well as how to gracefully and confidently make your way through the maze of your thoughts and emotions. We'll talk about the value of good nutrition, physical activity, and rest in fostering a strong physical frame that can carry you through life's adventures. We'll also explore spirituality and look at how it contributes to inner serenity, meaning, and purpose.

As you read the eBook, you'll discover helpful exercises, true accounts of people who have changed their lives for the better via holistic self-care, and priceless resources to support you along the way. The aim is to empower you to create a sustainable and enriching self-care routine tailored to your unique needs and aspirations.

A NEW BEGINNING

Here is where your path to holistic self-care begins. Self-love, self-compassion, and self-discovery are all steps along the route. It's a recognition that you merit more than just survival—you deserve to thrive. It's an invitation to live in the richness of who you are and to set out on a journey to equilibrium, energy, and a closer relationship with both yourself and the world around you.

Are you prepared to start this life-changing journey? Let's start.

CHAPTER 1
Understanding Holistic Self-Care

The idea of self-care has become quite popular in today's society and is frequently associated with decadent activities like spa days, bubble baths, and splurges. Even while these activities might be relaxing, true self-care entails a profound dedication to fostering your complete well-being. In this chapter, we'll examine the fundamentals of comprehensive self-care and explain why it forms the basis of a happy existence.

DEFINING HOLISTIC SELF-CARE

A paradigm shift that acknowledges the intricate and unbreakable relationship between your mind, body, and spirit is what holistic self-care is more than simply a trend. It embraces the notion that these facets of your personality are intertwined, and taking care of one has an immediate impact on the others. Let's examine what each of these elements implies in more detail:

- **Mind:** Your mind is the epicenter of your thoughts, emotions, and consciousness. It's the part of you that experiences joy, sorrow, inspiration, and stress. Holistic self-care for the mind involves practices that promote mental clarity, emotional resilience, and inner peace.

- **Body:** Your body is your physical vessel—the magnificent machine that carries you through life's adventures. It requires proper nourishment, exercise, and rest to function optimally. Holistic self-care for the body encompasses nutrition, fitness, and sleep hygiene, among other factors.

- **Spirit:** Your spirit represents the essence of your inner self—the part of you that seeks meaning, purpose, and connection. It's the source of your values and beliefs. Holistic self-care for the spirit involves nurturing your sense of purpose, exploring spirituality, and fostering a deep inner connection.

THE INTERCONNECTEDNESS OF MIND, BODY, AND SPIRIT

Imagine your mind, body, and spirit as three threads in a delicate tapestry, each thread influencing and supporting the others. When one thread is pulled, the entire tapestry is affected. This interconnectedness is at the heart of holistic self-care. Consider these examples:

- **Stress:** Chronic stress can wreak havoc on both your mind and body. It can lead to anxiety, depression, and other mental health issues. Physically, stress triggers the release of hormones that can harm your cardiovascular system and weaken your immune system.

- **Exercise:** Engaging in regular physical activity not only strengthens your body but also boosts your mood and enhances mental clarity. It can be a spiritual practice, too, by allowing you to connect with your body and the present moment.

- **Meditation:** Mindfulness meditation is a practice that calms the mind, reduces stress, and fosters emotional resilience. It's often deeply spiritual, helping individuals connect with their inner selves and the universe.

WHY HOLISTIC SELF-CARE MATTERS

The modern lifestyle can often be overwhelming, leaving us mentally drained, physically exhausted, and spiritually disconnected. Neglecting any one aspect of ourselves can lead to imbalance and discontent. Holistic self-care matters because it offers a solution to these challenges.

By embracing holistic self-care, you'll:

- Experience greater overall well-being and life satisfaction.
- Learn to manage stress and navigate life's challenges with resilience.
- Foster a deeper connection with yourself, your values, and your purpose.
- Enhance your physical health, energy, and vitality.
- Cultivate a profound sense of inner peace and contentment.

THE JOURNEY AHEAD

In the chapters that follow, we'll explore each dimension of holistic self-care in detail, providing practical insights and actionable strategies for nurturing your mind, body, and spirit. You'll learn how to integrate these practices into your daily life, creating a personalized self-care routine that empowers you to thrive.

Are you ready to embark on this journey of holistic self-care? Let's begin with the mind in Chapter 2, where we'll delve into mindfulness and stress management techniques.

CHAPTER 2
Nurturing Your Mind

Your mind is a powerful instrument, the epicenter of your thoughts, emotions, and consciousness. It's where creativity flourishes, where you make decisions, and where you experience the world. In this chapter, we'll explore the essential components of holistic self-care for the mind, delving into mindfulness, stress management, emotional resilience, and the practices that lead to a clearer and more peaceful mental landscape.

MINDFULNESS MEDITATION TECHNIQUES

Mindfulness is the practice of being fully present in the moment, observing your thoughts and feelings without judgment. It's a transformative practice that can significantly impact your mental well-being. Here are some mindfulness meditation techniques to get you started:

1. **Breath Awareness Meditation:** Focus on your breath as you inhale and exhale. Notice the sensations of each breath without trying to change them. This practice cultivates mindfulness and calms the mind.

2. **Body Scan Meditation:** Progressively bring your awareness to each part of your body, starting from your toes and moving up to your head. Notice any tension or sensations, and allow them to dissolve as you bring awareness to them.

3. **Loving-Kindness Meditation (Metta):** Send wishes of love, kindness, and compassion to yourself, loved ones, and even those you may have conflicts with. This practice promotes emotional well-being and empathy.

4. **Walking Meditation:** Practice mindfulness while walking. Pay attention to each step, the sensation of your feet lifting and touching the ground, and the sounds and sights around you.

STRESS MANAGEMENT STRATEGIES

Stress is a common companion in our lives, and managing it effectively is crucial for mental well-being. Here are some stress management strategies:

1. **Deep Breathing Exercises:** Practice deep breathing to activate the body's relaxation response. Inhale deeply through your nose, hold for a moment, and exhale slowly through your mouth. Repeat several times.

2. **Progressive Muscle Relaxation:** Tense and release different muscle groups to relieve physical tension associated with stress.

3. **Journaling:** Write down your thoughts and emotions to gain clarity and reduce mental clutter. It can also help identify sources of stress.

4. **Time Management:** Organize your tasks, prioritize them, and break them into manageable chunks. Avoid overloading your schedule.

CULTIVATING EMOTIONAL RESILIENCE

Emotional resilience is the ability to bounce back from adversity and maintain mental and emotional well-being in the face of challenges. To cultivate emotional resilience:

1. **Practice Self-Compassion:** Treat yourself with kindness and understanding, especially during difficult times. Avoid self-criticism.

2. **Seek Support:** Talk to friends, family, or a mental health professional when needed. Sharing your thoughts and feelings can be immensely healing.

3. **Positive Self-Talk:** Challenge negative thought patterns and replace them with positive, empowering ones.

4. **Mindful Acceptance:** Practice acceptance of situations you cannot change. Focus on what you can control.

ENHANCING COGNITIVE WELLNESS

Cognitive wellness involves maintaining mental sharpness, memory, and cognitive abilities throughout life. Strategies to enhance cognitive wellness include:

1. **Lifelong Learning:** Continuously challenge your mind with new information, skills, and experiences.

2. **Brain-Boosting Nutrition:** Consume a diet rich in brain-boosting nutrients, including omega-3 fatty acids, antioxidants, and vitamins.

3. **Physical Activity:** Regular exercise not only benefits the body but also supports cognitive health by increasing blood flow to the brain.

4. **Adequate Sleep:** Prioritize quality sleep, as it plays a vital role in memory consolidation and cognitive function.

Incorporating these practices into your life can foster a clearer, more resilient mind that is better equipped to navigate life's challenges and embrace its joys. In the next chapter, we'll explore holistic self-care for the body, including nutrition, exercise, and rest.

CHAPTER 3
Caring for Your Body

Your body is a marvelous and sophisticated tool that serves as your window to the outside world. It is capable of amazing feats, but in order for it to operate at its best, it also needs care and attention. The essential elements of holistic self-care for the body, such as nutrition, exercise, sleep, and rituals that support physical vitality, will be discussed in this chapter.

NUTRITION FOR HOLISTIC HEALTH

Nutrition is the foundation of physical well-being and plays a significant role in your overall health. A balanced and mindful approach to nutrition can:

- **Boost Energy:** Provide the essential nutrients your body needs for sustained energy throughout the day.
- **Support Immunity:** Strengthen your immune system to ward off illnesses and infections.
- **Promote Digestive Health:** Foster a healthy gut microbiome for better digestion and nutrient absorption.
- **Maintain Weight:** Help you achieve and maintain a healthy weight, which is essential for overall health.

Consider these principles for mindful nutrition:

1. **Balanced Diet:** Consume a variety of foods from different food groups, emphasizing fruits, vegetables, whole grains, lean proteins, and healthy fats.
2. **Portion Control:** Be mindful of portion sizes to avoid overeating and support a healthy weight.
3. **Hydration:** Drink an adequate amount of water daily to stay hydrated and support bodily functions.
4. **Mindful Eating:** Practice eating mindfully, savoring each bite, and paying attention to hunger and fullness cues.
5. **Limit Processed Foods:** Reduce consumption of highly

processed and sugary foods, which can lead to health issues.

PHYSICAL ACTIVITY AND EXERCISE

Regular physical activity is not only essential for maintaining physical health but also plays a crucial role in mental and emotional well-being. Benefits of physical activity include:

- **Strength and Endurance:** Building strength and endurance to perform daily activities with ease.
- **Mood Enhancement:** Releasing endorphins that boost mood and reduce stress.
- **Weight Management:** Supporting a healthy weight and reducing the risk of chronic diseases.
- **Cardiovascular Health:** Enhancing heart health and improving blood circulation.

Consider incorporating these elements into your physical activity routine:

1. **Aerobic Exercise:** Engage in activities such as walking, jogging, swimming, or dancing to improve cardiovascular health.

2. **Strength Training:** Include strength training exercises using weights or resistance bands to build and maintain muscle mass.

3. **Flexibility and Balance:** Practice activities like yoga or tai chi to improve flexibility and balance, reducing the risk of injuries.

4. **Consistency:** Aim for regular physical activity, striving to achieve at least 150 minutes of moderate-intensity

aerobic activity per week.

QUALITY SLEEP FOR VITALITY

Sleep is a fundamental component of holistic self-care. It is during sleep that your body and mind undergo essential processes for restoration and rejuvenation. Quality sleep can:

- **Boost Cognitive Function:** Enhance memory, problem-solving, and overall cognitive performance.

- **Support Emotional Well-Being:** Improve mood regulation and emotional resilience.

- **Aid Physical Recovery:** Promote tissue repair, muscle growth, and immune system functioning.

To promote healthy sleep:

1. **Create a Sleep-Friendly Environment:** Ensure your bedroom is comfortable, dark, and quiet. Consider using white noise machines or earplugs if necessary.

2. **Establish a Sleep Routine:** Go to bed and wake up at the same time each day, even on weekends.

3. **Limit Screen Time:** Avoid electronic devices with bright screens at least an hour before bedtime, as the blue light can interfere with sleep.

4. **Mindful Relaxation:** Engage in relaxation techniques, such as deep breathing or meditation, to calm the mind before sleep.

HOLISTIC WELLNESS PRACTICES

In addition to nutrition, physical activity, and sleep, holistic self-care for the body includes practices such as:

- **Hygiene:** Maintain personal hygiene to promote physical health and well-being.

- **Massage and Bodywork:** Consider massage therapy or other bodywork techniques to relieve tension and support relaxation.

- **Breathing Exercises:** Practice deep breathing exercises to reduce stress and enhance lung capacity.

- **Regular Health Checkups:** Schedule regular checkups with healthcare professionals to monitor your overall health.

By nurturing your body through mindful nutrition, regular physical activity, quality sleep, and holistic wellness practices, you can support your physical vitality and create a solid foundation for holistic well-being. In the next chapter, we'll explore holistic self-care for the spirit, including the role of spirituality and practices that connect you with your inner self.

CHAPTER 4
Feeding Your Spirit

The part of you that looks for meaning, purpose and a connection to something more than yourself is known as your spirit. In this chapter, we'll examine the significance of spirituality, the mind-body-spirit link, finding purpose and meaning, and holistic spiritual activities that enhance your inner world. Spirituality is a crucial component of holistic self-care.

SPIRITUALITY AND ITS ROLE IN SELF-CARE

Religion has no bearing on the extremely subjective and individualistic experience of spirituality. It includes a sense of kinship with the cosmos, a quest for meaning, and an investigation into the secrets of life. Adopting a spiritual outlook can:

- **Provide Meaning and Purpose:** Help you discover a sense of purpose and direction in your life.
- **Foster Inner Peace:** Bring a sense of tranquility and contentment.
- **Enhance Resilience:** Offer support during challenging times and provide a framework for understanding suffering.
- **Promote Empathy:** Encourage compassion and understanding for others.

MIND-BODY-SPIRIT CONNECTION

The mind, body, and spirit are intricately connected, and holistic self-care recognizes this unity. Consider the following aspects of the mind-body-spirit connection:

1. **Emotions and Physical Health:** Emotional well-being can significantly impact physical health. Chronic stress, for example, can lead to physical health issues.

2. **Spirituality and Mental Health:** Exploring your spirituality can enhance your mental health by providing a sense of purpose and inner peace.

3. **Mindful Practices:** Practices like meditation and yoga bridge the gap between the mind, body, and spirit, promoting overall well-being.

4. **Holistic Healing:** Holistic therapies often address the interconnectedness of the mind, body, and spirit in the healing process.

FINDING MEANING AND PURPOSE

A sense of meaning and purpose is a powerful driver of well-being. To discover or deepen your sense of purpose:

- **Reflect on Values:** Consider your core values and beliefs and how they align with your daily life.

- **Set Meaningful Goals:** Pursue goals and activities that resonate with your sense of purpose.

- **Connect with Passion:** Engage in activities you are passionate about, as they often align with your sense of purpose.

- **Contribute to Others:** Helping others and contributing to a greater cause can provide a profound sense of purpose.

EXPLORING HOLISTIC SPIRITUAL PRACTICES

Holistic spiritual practices are diverse and adaptable to individual beliefs and preferences. Some practices to explore include:

1. **Meditation:** Mindfulness meditation and guided meditation can connect you with your inner self and the present moment.

2. **Yoga:** Yoga is not just a physical practice; it also encompasses breath work and meditation, fostering a mind-body-spirit connection.

3. **Nature Connection:** Spending time in nature can be a spiritual experience, allowing you to connect with the world around you.

4. **Journaling:** Reflect on your spiritual journey through journaling, exploring your thoughts, experiences, and insights.

5. **Community and Rituals:** Engage in spiritual communities or rituals that resonate with your beliefs and values.

6. **Prayer and Affirmations:** Spiritual practices like prayer and positive affirmations can strengthen your connection with your inner self and a higher power.

EMBRACING HOLISTIC SPIRITUALITY

Holistic self-care for the spirit is about embracing the uniqueness of your spiritual journey. It's about recognizing that your path may differ from others and that your beliefs and practices are deeply personal. As you continue your journey of self-care, remember that nourishing your spirit is a vital component of your holistic well-being.

In the next chapter, we will explore how to integrate holistic self-care into your daily life. We'll provide guidance on creating a personalized self-care routine that encompasses the mind, body, and spirit, empowering you to thrive in all aspects of your life.

CHAPTER 5
Integrating Holistic Self-Care into Your Daily Life

Embracing holistic self-care is not a one-time event but a continuous journey toward overall well-being. It's about weaving mindful practices into your daily life to nurture your mind, body, and spirit consistently. In this chapter, we'll explore how to create a holistic self-care routine, set SMART self-care goals, overcome common challenges, and adapt self-care to busy lifestyles.

CREATING A HOLISTIC SELF-CARE ROUTINE

A holistic self-care routine is a personalized and sustainable set of practices that nourish your mind, body, and spirit. Here's how to create one:

1. **Assess Your Needs:** Reflect on what aspects of your well-being require attention. Consider your mental, emotional, physical, and spiritual needs.

2. **Choose Practices:** Select practices that resonate with you. They should align with your goals and preferences.

3. **Set a Schedule:** Determine when and how often you'll engage in self-care practices. Consistency is key.

4. **Start Small:** Begin with a few practices and gradually expand as you become more comfortable.

5. **Mindful Awareness:** Approach your routine with mindfulness and presence, fully engaging in each practice.

SETTING SMART SELF-CARE GOALS

Effective self-care is goal-oriented and purposeful. SMART goals (Specific, Measurable, Achievable, Relevant, and Time-bound) can guide your self-care journey:

- **Specific:** Clearly define your self-care goal. For example, "I will practice mindfulness meditation for 10 minutes every morning."

- **Measurable:** Set criteria to track your progress. In the case of meditation, you could measure the number of days you meditate each week.

- **Achievable:** Ensure your goal is realistic and attainable. Starting with 10 minutes of meditation daily may be more achievable than an hour.

- **Relevant:** Your goal should align with your holistic well-being. For instance, improving sleep quality is relevant to overall health.

- **Time-bound:** Set a timeline for achieving your goal. "I will establish a consistent meditation practice within the next 30 days."

OVERCOMING COMMON CHALLENGES

Holistic self-care may face obstacles, but acknowledging and addressing these challenges can help you stay on track:

1. **Time Constraints:** Prioritize self-care by scheduling it into your day. Even short practices can make a difference.

2. **Lack of Motivation:** Start with practices you enjoy to boost motivation. Consider setting small rewards for achieving self-care goals.

3. **Overcommitment:** Avoid overloading your self-care routine. Keep it manageable and adaptable.

4. **Inconsistency:** If you miss a day or practice, don't be discouraged. Gentle self-compassion can help you get back on track.

5. **Negative Self-Talk:** Replace self-criticism with positive affirmations and self-encouragement.

SELF-CARE FOR BUSY LIFESTYLES

In today's fast-paced world, busy schedules can make self-care seem elusive. However, with adaptability and creativity, self-care can still be integrated into your life:

1. **Micro-Moments of Self-Care:** Find small pockets of time for brief self-care practices. This could be a few minutes of deep breathing during a work break or a short nature walk.

2. **Prioritize Self-Care:** Recognize the importance of self-care for your overall well-being and make it a non-negotiable part of your routine.

3. **Delegate and Seek Support:** Share responsibilities with others and ask for support when needed. This can free up time for self-care.

4. **Batch Tasks:** Consolidate tasks to create more free time for self-care. For example, prepare meals for the week in advance to save cooking time.

5. **Learn to Say No:** Set boundaries and prioritize self-care by declining commitments that overwhelm you.

EMBRACE SELF-CARE AS A LIFESTYLE

Holistic self-care is not a checklist of activities but a way of life. It's a commitment to nurturing your mind, body, and spirit consistently, recognizing that your well-being is a valuable and ongoing journey.

As you embark on this journey, remember that self-care is a deeply personal experience. What works for one person may not work for another. Embrace the practices that resonate with you, adapt them to your unique needs, and allow self-care to be a source of empowerment and enrichment in your life.

In the next chapter, we'll explore inspiring stories of individuals who have transformed their lives through holistic self-care, illustrating the profound impact it can have.

CHAPTER 6
Holistic Self-Care Success Stories

We have looked at the many facets of holistic self-care in the pages that follow; we have delved into the mind, body, and spirit; and we have learned how to incorporate these practices into daily life. It's time to hear from those who have started their own holistic self-care journeys and have seen amazing changes along the way.

INSPIRING STORIES OF TRANSFORMATION

1. Sarah's Journey to Mindful Living

Sarah, a marketing executive, was accustomed to the fast-paced demands of her career. She often felt overwhelmed and struggled with anxiety. After experiencing burnout, she decided to explore holistic self-care. She started practicing mindfulness meditation daily, even if it was just for a few minutes. Gradually, she noticed a significant reduction in her stress levels. Mindfulness gave her the ability to stay calm under pressure and improved her focus at work. Sarah's journey to mindful living not only transformed her work-life balance but also enhanced her overall well-being.

2. Jake's Transformation through Physical Wellness

Jake, a software engineer, had a sedentary lifestyle and often felt sluggish. He decided to prioritize physical wellness. Jake began with short daily walks and gradually incorporated strength training exercises. Over time, he gained more energy, shed excess weight, and improved his self-esteem. What started as a quest for better physical health evolved into a passion for fitness. Jake now participates in marathons and encourages his colleagues to adopt healthier habits. His journey is a testament to the transformative power of physical self-care.

3. Ella's Spiritual Awakening

Ella, a stay-at-home mom, felt a void in her life despite having a loving family. She began exploring spirituality, attending meditation classes, and connecting with like-minded individuals.

This journey led her to a profound spiritual awakening. Ella discovered a deep sense of purpose and inner peace, which positively influenced her family life. She introduced her children to mindfulness practices, creating a more harmonious and spiritually connected household.

THE IMPACT ON THEIR LIVES

These stories are not isolated instances but representative of the profound transformations that holistic self-care can bring:

- Sarah found inner peace and improved her professional life.
- Jake experienced a physical and mental transformation that elevated his confidence.
- Ella discovered a deep sense of purpose and shared the benefits of her journey with her family.

These stories illustrate that holistic self-care is not just a concept but a life-changing journey that can empower individuals to thrive in various aspects of their lives.

YOUR JOURNEY AWAITS

You have learned more about the comprehensive approach to self-care as you have read this eBook's pages. You've studied how to design a tailored self-care schedule and have looked into practices that support your mind, body, and soul.

It's time for you to start your own trip right now. Keep in mind that every person has an own path to holistic self-care, which may change over time. Self-care has the ability to transform, so embrace it and be patient with yourself.

In the final chapter of this eBook, we will provide you with valuable resources to support your holistic self-care journey, including recommended books, online communities, mindfulness apps, and professional guidance.

CHAPTER 7
Resources for Your Holistic Self-Care Journey

Your holistic self-care journey is a personal and transformative exploration of your mind, body, and spirit. To support you on this journey, we've compiled a wealth of resources, from recommended books and further reading to online communities, mindfulness and wellness apps, and professional guidance.

RECOMMENDED BOOKS AND FURTHER READING

1. *The Miracle of Mindfulness* by Thich Nhat Hanh
   - This classic book introduces mindfulness meditation and offers practical guidance on integrating mindfulness into daily life.

2. *The Body Keeps the Score* by Bessel van der Kolk
   - Explore the connection between trauma, the body, and healing. This book delves into the impact of trauma on the body and mind and provides insights into holistic healing.

3. *The Power of Now* by Eckhart Tolle
   - Eckhart Tolle's teachings on the present moment and spiritual awakening have resonated with millions. Discover a deeper understanding of consciousness and self.

4. *The Plant-Based Solution* by Joel K. Kahn, MD
   - Explore the benefits of a plant-based diet for physical well-being. This book provides insights into nutrition and heart health.

5. *Radical Acceptance* by Tara Brach
   - Tara Brach offers a path to self-compassion and self-acceptance. Learn how to embrace yourself with love and understanding.

ONLINE COMMUNITIES AND SUPPORT

1. **Reddit's r/Mindfulness and r/Meditation:**
   - Engage in discussions, share experiences, and learn from a global community of mindfulness and meditation enthusiasts.

2. **Goodreads Self-Help and Self-Improvement Groups:**
   - Join online book clubs and discussions focused on self-care, personal growth, and well-being.

3. **Meetup.com:**
   - Explore local and online groups and events centered around holistic self-care practices, such as meditation groups or wellness workshops.

Mindfulness and Wellness Apps

1. **Headspace:**
   - A popular mindfulness app that offers guided meditation sessions, sleep stories, and mindfulness exercises.

2. **Calm:**
   - Calm provides meditation, relaxation, and sleep aid content, including guided meditation sessions and soothing sounds.

3. **Insight Timer:**
   - This app offers a vast library of free guided meditations and mindfulness practices led by

experienced teachers.

4. **MyFitnessPal:**
   - Track your nutrition and physical activity, helping you maintain a balanced diet and active lifestyle.

PROFESSIONAL GUIDANCE AND SERVICES

1. **Therapy and Counseling:**
   - Consider seeking the guidance of a licensed therapist or counselor for mental health support and emotional well-being.

2. **Nutritionists and Dietitians:**
   - Consult with a registered dietitian or nutritionist for personalized dietary guidance and meal planning.

3. **Personal Trainers and Fitness Instructors:**
   - If you're new to exercise or want tailored fitness routines, a personal trainer or fitness instructor can provide expert guidance.

4. **Spiritual and Holistic Practitioners:**
   - Connect with practitioners who specialize in holistic therapies like acupuncture, energy healing, or Reiki.

Remember that your holistic self-care journey is uniquely yours. These resources are here to support and enrich your path, but the choices you make along the way are guided by your personal needs and preferences. Embrace the power of self-care, and may your journey be one of continued growth, balance, and well-being.

CONCLUSION
A Holistic Path to Well-Being

Greetings, you have completed "Holistic Self-Care: Balancing Mind, Body, and Spirit." This path of self-discovery, empowerment, and transformation has taken place within the domains of the mind, body, and spirit. Let's think about the fundamentals of comprehensive self-care and how important it is to our lives as we draw to a conclusion this eBook.

THE WHOLENESS OF HOLISTIC SELF-CARE

Holistic self-care is a way of life—an intentional decision to embrace the entirety of who you are. It is not a single practice or a passing fad. It recognizes that you are a complex tapestry of many factors woven together, not just your thoughts, body, or beliefs. You take care of the foundations of your wellbeing when you take care of your mind, body, and spirit.

A TAPESTRY OF WELL-BEING

You have studied the practice of mindfulness, stress reduction, and mental emotional toughness throughout these chapters. You've studied the relationship between your body's need for rest and your diet, exercise, and other activities. You've started a spiritual journey in search of meaning, connection, and a reason for your existence. You've mastered incorporating these routines into your life to create a self-care regimen that enables you to flourish.

THE TRANSFORMATIVE POWER OF SELF-CARE

You've heard moving tales of people who used holistic self-care to completely change their lives. These experiences serve as a reminder that self-care is a valuable skill that is available to everyone, not just the wealthy. Holistic self-care can help you reach your objectives, whether they are inner tranquility, physical vitality, or a greater sense of purpose.

A PERSONAL JOURNEY

Your holistic self-care journey is uniquely yours. It may involve meditation or yoga, a plant-based diet or regular exercise, spiritual exploration or artistic expression. Your journey may ebb and flow, adapting to the seasons of your life. What matters most is your commitment to yourself and your well-being.

A LIFELONG COMMITMENT

As you close the pages of this eBook, remember that your journey doesn't end here; it's an ongoing commitment to your well-being. It's a promise to nurture your mind, body, and spirit throughout the chapters of your life. It's an acknowledgment that you deserve to thrive, not just survive.

EMBRACE SELF-CARE AS A WAY OF LIFE

Holistic self-care is not a checklist but a way of life. It's a choice to embrace the fullness of your existence, to care for yourself with love and intention, and to honor the interconnectedness of your mind, body, and spirit. It's a reminder that you are worthy of the time and attention you invest in yourself.

YOUR HOLISTIC SELF-CARE JOURNEY CONTINUES

As you navigate the intricate dance of your mind, body, and spirit, remember that you are not alone. Seek support when needed, explore new practices, and adapt to the ever-evolving landscape of your well-being. Your journey is a continuous exploration, an ongoing quest for balance, vitality, and fulfillment.

THE POWER OF SELF-CARE IN THE WORLD

As you thrive through holistic self-care, you radiate positivity and well-being into the world around you. Your self-care journey has a ripple effect, influencing your relationships, your community, and ultimately, the world. By nurturing yourself, you contribute to the collective well-being of humanity.

THANK YOU FOR THIS JOURNEY

Thank you for embarking on this journey of holistic self-care with us. May your path be filled with moments of self-discovery, growth, and transformation. May you embrace the fullness of your being and thrive in every aspect of your life. Your well-being matters, and your journey continues—one mindful, balanced, and spirited step at a time.

With love and well wishes on your holistic self-care journey.

Chimezie Igwe

APPENDIX
Additional Resources

In this section, you'll find a compilation of additional resources to further support your holistic self-care journey. These resources include recommended reading, online courses, and websites that offer valuable information and tools for your well-being.

BOOKS FOR CONTINUED LEARNING

1. *The Mindful Path to Self-Compassion* by Christopher K. Germer, PhD
   - A guide to cultivating self-compassion and resilience through mindfulness practices.

2. *Holistic Wellness in The New Age* by Dr. Anita Bhandari
   - Explores holistic wellness through a combination of traditional and modern approaches.

3. *The Four Agreements: A Practical Guide to Personal Freedom* by Don Miguel Ruiz
   - Offers insights into personal growth and transformation through ancient Toltec wisdom.

ONLINE COURSES AND WORKSHOPS

1. **Coursera** (www.coursera.org):
    - Offers a wide range of courses on mindfulness, well-being, nutrition, and more from top universities and institutions.

2. **Udemy** (www.udemy.com):
    - Provides affordable courses on various self-care topics, including meditation, yoga, and stress management.

3. **Mindful Schools** (www.mindfulschools.org):
    - Offers online courses and resources for educators, parents, and individuals interested in mindfulness.

WEBSITES AND BLOGS

1. **Mindful.org** (www.mindful.org):
     - A comprehensive resource for mindfulness practices, articles, and guided meditations.

2. **NutritionFacts.org** (www.nutritionfacts.org):
     - Provides evidence-based information on nutrition and its impact on health.

3. **Psychology Today** (www.psychologytoday.com):
     - Features articles, blogs, and directories of mental health professionals to support your well-being.

WELLNESS APPS

1. **Gratitude Journal - Happyfeed:**
   - Encourages daily gratitude practice and journaling for increased well-being.

2. **MyPlate by Livestrong:**
   - Helps track your nutrition, set health goals, and improve your diet.

3. **Fitbod:**
   - Offers personalized workout plans and fitness tracking for a well-rounded physical self-care routine.

PROFESSIONAL GUIDANCE

1. **American Psychological Association** (www.apa.org):
   - Provides resources for finding a psychologist or therapist for mental health support.

2. **Academy of Nutrition and Dietetics** (www.eatright.org):
   - Offers guidance on finding a registered dietitian for personalized nutrition advice.

3. **Yoga Alliance** (www.yogaalliance.org):
   - Helps you locate certified yoga instructors and studios for your yoga practice.

Note: Please verify the credibility and suitability of any resources or professionals before engaging with them. Your well-being is of utmost importance.

These additional resources are intended to complement your holistic self-care journey and provide you with options for further exploration and support. Remember that self-care is a dynamic and evolving process, and you have the power to shape it according to your unique needs and aspirations.

ACKNOWLEDGMENT

As I finish authoring this eBook on "Holistic Self-Care: Balancing Mind, Body, and Spirit," I am incredibly grateful for all of the encouragement, wisdom, and guidance that have helped me along the way.

I want to start by expressing my sincere gratitude to everyone who offered their personal narratives, firsthand knowledge, and unique perspectives on holistic self-care. Your generosity and openness have improved this eBook and increased its relatability and authenticity.

I would want to express my gratitude to all of the writers, educators, and practitioners whose works have served as a source of information and inspiration. The content of this eBook has benefited greatly from your contributions to the disciplines of mindfulness, nutrition, fitness, spirituality, and wellbeing.

I want to express my gratitude to my family and friends for their continuous support and inspiration. Your commitment to holistic health and self-care has served as a regular reminder of the value of this subject.

I owe a great deal of gratitude to the staff at [Your Publishing Platform], whose knowledge and direction made the production of this eBook a simple and satisfying task.

Finally, I would like to express my sincere gratitude to the readers of this eBook. The reason why sharing this information is so meaningful is because of your curiosity and dedication to self-care. I hope the ideas and methods you've learned about here will be helpful resources for you as you embark on a holistic self-care journey.

I wish you health, harmony, and further growth on your journey. I appreciate you being with me on this exploration of holistic self-care.

With warm regards,